I0413121

Hammer Lane

7 Lessons on How to Eat Healthier On the Road, Even though you're 'BUSY'... so you can drive more miles!

By

Sakani D'Angeles

Copyright © 2015 by DBC GLOBAL, INC.

ALL RIGHTS RESERVED

ISBN-13: 978-1495938603

Edition: b4hj

Note:
DBC PUBLISHING GLOBAL, INC. does not allow for this document, in its present form and with no alterations, to be distributed, printed, photocopied, reproduced, and/or disbursed by electronic means for the purpose of spreading its content and not for the purpose of gaining a profit, unless a specific request is sent to the publishers and permission is granted. Anyone wishing to quote from this document must give credit to the publisher.

Thank you for reading this book.

SUPPORT THE TEACHERS WHO TEACH BENEFICIAL INFORMATION THAT HELP PEOPLE IMPROVE-

5% of all author royalties are donated to educational not-for-profits.

If you choose to follow the information in this book that is based on scientific proof and practical application among many people then you should achieve the results you wish for.

If you decide to alter what is in this book and you get results other than what you are looking for then you are keeping yourself from

driving more miles.

Waiver of Liability
The meal & exercise information provided in this book is believed to be authentic & accurate based on the best judgment of the author. The reader is responsible for consulting with their own health or fitness professional on any matters raised within the book. Health information changes rapidly. I do not assume any liability for the information contained within this book, be it direct, indirect, consequential, special, exemplary, or other damages.

Before changing your exercise program please consult your physician. Any & all product names referenced within this book are copyright and trademarks of their respective owner.

CONTENTS

INTRODUCTION
WHO KNOWS?
WHAT IS HAMMER LANE?

PART 1
MEAL PLAN

PART 2
7 LESSONS

AFTER WAKING UP
ENOUGH EATING?
DINNER TIME?
VITAMINS ANYONE?
ENERGY UP!
TIME BETWEEN STOPS?
MOST IMPORTANT FOR ENERGY?

Conclusion
Acknowledgments

INTRODUCTION

My name is Sakani (sa-connie) D'Angeles. Author of this book and 5 other healthy eating and exercising books available on Barnes & Noble's website: www.bn.com. I am Coach of flowologee. It is an healthy eating and exercising program designed for 'BUSY' Professionals whether they think they have time or not.

I have tested and have lived by the principles you will learn in this book since 2003. I also was a Professional, Over the Road, 48 state Truck Driver and ate the way you will learn with the limited options on the highways of America. I also exercised the way you will learn with the limited space and equipment.

My program was effective before I started Truck Driving in 2006. The truck driving experience forced me to adjust my program and cut away what is really necessary in a eating and workout program: basic principles that can be adapted no matter what food is available and an exercise program stripped down to the basics the do not take too much time.

Time is the most important asset on the road for a Truck Driver and so is **rest**. The challenge was how to adapt my eating method and exercise method to the hard life on the road.

And that is the problem...

How can a Professional Over the Road Driver stay healthy while their 'BUSY' and without wearing themselves out in the process?

3 words: Read this book

Who Knows?

Dr. Williams Sheppard, D.C., of Katy, TX examined me twice during the creation of the first draft of this book for the official Department of Transportation Physical required of CDL holders for Knight Transportation. He was impressed the first time and was impressed with my improved results again months later when I took a second physical.

You picked up this book because you want to be healthier on the road. I respectfully suggest you keep an open mind to the concepts, strategies, tactics and basic principles outlined in this book.

If you do what is in this book to the best of your ability you should have excellent improvement, sleep better, feel better, and drive more miles which means more money for you and your family.

To better levels of fitness and more miles,

Sakani D'Angeles

What is Hammer Lane?

As you already know Hammer Lane is the fast lane. Why did I name this book Hammer Lane? I named it this way because the eating method I teach in this book along with the exercises helped me stay healthy on the road and that equaled in driving more miles. The info in this book should help you in the hammer lane.

Why is there a need for Hammer Lane?

I was a Professional Over the Road 48 State Truck Driver. I have been to every state except Montana, New Hampshire, Maine and Vermont. I have been on almost every major highway in America and I know what the life is like out there. Increasing rules from The Department of Transportation and from Trucking companies has made being healthy a very big issue. It should be and not because of the newer rules. It should be because for most Drivers there is someone at home waiting on them to return and to come home safe.

The healthier a Driver the better they can perform. It is all about what we Drivers do to take care of our families.

Eating the way I shall teach you in this book should also help you NOT be so exhausted on your days off so you can spend time with your family, etc.

The reality of our life when it comes to seeking good health is that there are

2 types of people:

Opportunity Health Seekers
Those people who buy every new 'diet' or workout program.

Strategic Health Thinkers
Those who 'think' about whether or not the new 'diet' or workout program **fits** in with how they are eating and exercising.

Be the **Strategic Health Thinker** because...

Poor strategy results in poor results

What does this mean to you as a Driver?

It means: The **ONLY** way to drive more miles, make more money, spend time with your family and be healthier is to be **'SMARTER / EFFECTIVE'** with your eating even with the limited eating choices on the road.

If I can do it with Subway, Denny's, Iron Skillet, etc...

You can too!

PART 1
Meal Plan & Dinner Examples

MEAL PLAN

MEAL PLAN

There **IS** a way to convert body fat into energy. I have complied and practiced a meal plan that has been around since the late 1800's. The details are beyond the scope of this book. Here we are doing 1 thing and 1 thing only...

We are using dinner to get your body used to converting body fat into energy. They way we do that is first understanding that dinner is the most important meal in converting body fat into energy / burning off the body fat.

So, the most important meal for the rest of your life for converting body fat into energy (losing body fat) is **DINNER**:

PROTEINS + VEGGIES
ONLY

This means: Chicken, Fish, Lamb, Goat, Steak whatever meat you like (we do not recommend pork) and vegetables ONLY. Ice cream is okay for desert.

QUICK FOOD LIST:

PROTEINS

BEANS-BBQ-BAKED BISON, CHICKEN BREAST-CHICKEN THIGH-EGG-FISH-LAMB-LENTILS-SHRIMP-TUNA WHITE-TURKEY, BREAST-VEAL CUTLET-WHITEFISH-TOFU, ETC.

PROTEINS
(DAIRY GROUP)

BUTTERMILK-CHEESE, AMERICAN, CHEDDAR, FET, MOZZARELLA, PARMESAN, SWISS-COTTAGE CHEESE-EGG WHITE, YOLK-HALF & HALF-MILK, SKIM, LOWFAT, 2%, WHOLE, SOUR CREAM-SOY MILK-WHIPPED CREAM-WHIPPING CREAM-YOGURT, PLAIN, NON-FAT, LOWFAT, ETC.

CARBOHYDRATES
BAGELS-BEANS-BREAD-CEREAL-CRACKERS-CORNBREAD-CREAM OF WHEAT-DANISH PASTRY-GRAHAM CRACKERS-HAMBURGER ROLL-MUFFIN-OATMEAL-PANCAKE-PASTA-POTATO-RICE-SWEET POTATO-TORTILLA-WAFFLE

OILS & FATS
OLIVE OIL-CORN OIL-AVOCADO-BUTTER-NUT OILS-SAFFLOWER OIL-SOY OIL SESAME OIL-CREAM, ETC.

VEGGIES
ASPARAGUS-BROCCOLI-BRUSSEL-CABBAGE-CARROTS-AULIFLOWER-CELERY-COLLARD GREENS-CORN ON THE COB-CORN-CUCUMBERS-EGGPLANT-GREEN BEANS-LETTUCE-MUSHROOMS-ONION-ONION RINGS-PEAS-PEPPERS-POTATOES-RADISHES-SPINACH-SQUASH-TOMATO, ALL VEGGIES, ETC.

FRUITS
APPLE/JUICE-APRICOT-AVOCADO-BANANA-BLACKBERRIES-CANTALOUPE-CRANBERRY/JUICE-FRUIT SALAD-GRAPEFRUIT-GRAPES-HONEY DEW MELON-KIWI-MANGO-ORANGE-ORANGE JUICE-PEACH-PEAR-PINEAPPLE/JUICE-PLUM-RAISINS-RED RASPBERRIES-STRAWBERRIES-WATERMELON,
ALL FRUITS, ETC.

MEAL PLAN
&
DINNER
EXAMPLES

DINNER ON THE ROAD:

PROTEINS + VEGGIES

ONLY

This means: Chicken, Fish, Lamb, Goat, Steak whatever meat you like (we do not recommend pork) and vegetables ONLY. Ice cream is okay for desert.

PROTEINS + VEGGIES

ONLY

This means: Chicken, Fish, Lamb, Goat, Steak whatever meat you like (we do not recommend pork) and vegetables ONLY. Ice cream is okay for desert.

DINNER EXAMPLES:

REMEMBER: THE CONCEPT IS PROTEINS + VEGGIES SO...

MEAL EXAMPLE #1:
V8 TOMATO JUICE + 8-12 OUNCE STEAK + BROCCOLLI

MEAL EXAMPLE #2:
CHICKEN BREAST + CARROTS & HALF OF A BAKED POTATO

MEAL EXAMPLE #3:
8-10 OUNCE BAKED FISH + MIXED VEGETABLES

MEAL EXAMPLE #4:
(YOUR NOT REALLY HUNGRY SO...)
2 CONTAINERS OF GREEK YOGURT

MEAL EXAMPLE #5:
LARGE TUNA FISH SALAD **WITHOUT** MAYO

REMEMBER HYDRATE = WATER, MILK, GATORADE, MINERAL WATER

PART 2

7 Lessons for Consistent Healthy Eating, Low
Body Fat and Increased Energy

AFTER WAKING UP

Traveling around America required I learn a more effective way to begin my day. Drinking coffee after waking up would lead me to a jittery rush of energy. I hoped to find a smoother way to wake up BEFORE drinking some coffee. I found that with **Lesson 1**.

I.

BEGIN YOUR DAY WITH A FRUIT PRE-BREAKFAST AND WAIT 30 MIN BEFORE EATING BREAKFAST

Natural sugars found in fruit are better than caffeine first thing in the morning.

Try a nice large cup of Apple Juice after you wake up and feel the great effect it will have on your morning!

It is also slow digesting so it will give you a prolonged feeling of energy instead of a jolt like most caffeine products do.

BEGIN YOUR DAY WITH A FRUIT PRE-BREAKFAST AND WAIT 30 MIN BEFORE EATING BREAKFAST

ENOUGH EATING?

Counting calories may be good for some people. That's not easy for Drivers on the road. The reality is most of us in America are not disciplined or focused enough to keep track of counting how much we eat throughout the day. That may have worked in the 90's.

Lesson 2 is the easiest way based and is over 1000 years old!

II.

SPLIT YOUR MEAL INTO 3 PARTS:
1=FOOD, 1=DRINK, 1=AIR
(Simple, effective portion control)

Split your stomach into 3 parts: 1 part for food. 1 part for air. 1 part for your drink. People living in deserts in many parts of the world have known the value of this easy eating for centuries.

Take a look at the portion sizes of Japanese and Traditional Chinese food to get an understanding of how to apply this! Using smaller plates and bowls will make this point easy to apply!

SPLIT YOUR MEAL INTO 3 PARTS:

DINNER TIME?

The body is a beautiful piece of organic machinery. It was designed immaculately and expertly. That said, the way to transform our bodies is to understand how it works. Fasting by abstaining from food or drink like when we go to sleep forces the body to use body fat as energy. Traveling also forced me to eat differently at dinner time because I needed to wake up early.

Too much food and NO ONE wakes up well!

Lesson 3 answers one of the best ways to convert body fat into energy.

III.
EAT NO CARBS FOR DINNER *NONE*

Your body needs carbs during the day as carbs are good fuel for the body.

Hugh Jackman of the Xmen movies admitted he was a believer in the golden rule of more frequent and smaller meals. He also followed this basic rule in preparing for Xmen Orgins: Wolverine and he said,

"I get up at 4am and eat egg whites, then every three hours after that... Then after midday, no ricc or carbohydrates. It's just vegetables and meat or fish."
(Showbiz: Comicbookmovie.com)

As you see in this story this is the best way to keep the body fat low. And body fat is the biggest issue with Drivers.

EAT NO CARBS FOR DINNER... MONDAY – FRIDAY *NONE*

VITMANS ANYONE?

If we all had farms or at least a little garden then it would be easier to eat fresh veggies. That said, we are not getting all that we need. Especially since we are working our bodies more and especially because Drivers do not eat enough vegetables. **Lesson 4** is a necessary tip.

IV.

TAKE A MULTIVITAMIN WITH BREAKFAST & DINNER

Most people do not take in enough vitamins to help their bodies while having busy schedules. Drivers again... don't eat enough vegetables.

A Boston Marathon runner told reminded me busy people need more vitamins than people who are not. And no doubt, most people in the 2000's are busier than ever.

TAKE A MULTIVITAMIN WITH BREAKFAST & DINNER

ENERGY UP?

It is known camping in Big Ben National Park, hiking through the Grand Canyon or traveling through any desert that if you DON'T hydrate you will become weak and your energy will sink.

Lesson 5 should be the most important of because of what the body is mostly made of.

V.

HYDRATE, HYDRATE, HYDRATE WITH MILK, WATER, GATORADE, ETC.

A review published in the Journal of the International Society of Sports Nutrition late last year found that drinking milk after exercise has positive effects on recovery, muscle building, and hydration. **(triathlete.com 12-8-2009)**

Of course, your not exercising. You are driving which is similar to exercising in that you are putting your body under stress while driving.

This is a challenge while driving. I suggest to hydrate through different sources: So sip gatorade, water, along with your offer drink throughout your drive time. When you shut down for the night then hydrate then: drink water, gatorade or milk then sleep.

You should sleep well and wake up hyrdated: full of water.

HYDRATE, HYDRATE, HYDRATE WITH MILK, WATER, GATORADE, ETC.

TIME BETWEEN STOPS?

Traveling again I was using up energy whether I was/am flying or driving. Flying I didn't feel the need to maintain a schedule. Driving was another story... If I didn't fill up my gas tank. I would run out of gas so **Lesson 6**...

VI.

EAT EVERY 3 TO 4 HOURS

Eating 5 meals a day with about 3-4 hours apart should ensure a steady flow of energy.

3 meals a day is no longer a practical way of eating considering the work schedules of many people is longer than 10 years ago.

EAT EVERY 3 TO 4 HOURS

MOST IMPORTANT FOR ENERGY?

The first cereal grains were domesticated over 8000 years ago. Ferdinand Schumacher, a German immigrant, began the cereals revolution in 1854 with a hand oats grinder in the back room of a small store in, Akron, Ohio. His German Mills American Oatmeal Company was the nation's first commercial oatmeal manufacturer. It was enough energy for thenm and then...

In a busier time like we live in we need more energy / more effective energy source first thing in the morning. **Lesson 7** is what I and many who travel and are very 'busy' have found to be the best. Try it and see!

VII.

MOST IMPORTANT MEALS FOR ENERGY

Breakfast is the most important meal to energize you for the day so remember: Breakfast foods like just cereal or oatmeal, etc. are no longer enough in the busy time we live in worldwide.

Eat a big breakfast as this should energize you for your day.

MOST IMPORTANT MEAL FOR ENERGY? EAT BIG BREAKFAST TO ENERGIZE YOUR DAY!

CONCLUSION

IMPORTANT TO REMEMBER:

MOST IMPORTANT MEAL FOR ENERGY IS:
BREAKFAST

MOST IMPORTANT MEAL FOR THE WAISTLINE IS:
DINNER

<u>DRINK ENOUGH</u>
MILK, WATER, GATORADE, MINERAL WATER, 100% JUICE

Acknowledgments...

First, I must thank **God** for the inspiration to teach this information that has keep and continues to keep me healthy and looking younger every day.

Thank you for having Mercy on me.

Dad & Mom
Always encouraging, top shelf, amazing parents who I am happy to have.
Ali Hakeem
Thanks for the support and being my little brother. Team work makes the dream work.
Yi-Chun Tricia Lin
Your inspiration and encouragement for me to write was a seed that I am glad you planted. I am honored to still have you in my life.

Everyone who I have met. Period. I am inspired by all.

Sakani D'Angeles

Special books or book excerpts can be created to fit specific needs.
For more information & details please email me: sakaniflowcoach@gmail.com

This book contains the complete text of the hardcover edition.

If you find any errors please email me at **sakaniflowcoach@gmail.com**

The meal & exercise information provided in this book is believed to be authentic & accurate based on the best judgment of the author.
The reader is responsible for consulting with their own health or fitness professional on any matters raised within the book.
Health information changes rapidly.
I do not assume any liability for the information contained within this book, be it direct, indirect, consequential, special, exemplary, or other damages.

Before changing your exercise program, please consult your physician. Any & all product names referenced within this book are **copyright and trademarks of their respective owner.**

Hammer Lane

7 Lessons on How to Eat Healthier On the Road, Even though you're 'BUSY'... so you can drive more miles!

By

Sakani D'Angeles

www.ingramcontent.com/pod-product-compliance
Lightning Source LLC
Chambersburg PA
CBHW080354290526

45791CB00009BA/2876